Eating It Up Right

BY Magalene Y. Noble

A Guide to a Healthier You

Table of content

To my children with all my love

Adam, Samantha, Matthew, Celeste

INTRODUCTION

Holy Toledo! Can't we all just get along? Oh I mean can't we all just eat right? I know, I know, for most of us easier said than done. Are you living to eat or are you eating to live? Sayings like that are sayings for a reason. We live in a world filled with great tasting food and a lot of it isn't very healthy for you, but it's not realistic to think you're just going to stay away from all that great tasting food. Believe me, I can't stay away from it, so I don't even try. I make sure I eat everything, I really do mean everything; pizza, hamburgers, eggs benedict, and Oysters Rockefeller. I eat to live, but I make sure I do more than just smell the coffee, if I'm eating out I'm going to enjoy the experience. When the holidays come around I do enjoy all food that's being made or baked and given to me.

I've been contemplating writing a book on how to stay slim, trim and most of all healthy for many years. I'm not a nutritionist or a dietitian but, I do pay attention to what the nutritionist have to say. This book is what I've learned over the years. A how to on making what you already know about eating easier without feeling hungry or like you have to deprive yourself. I'm a fifty two year old mother of four that has been thin all my life. But every day I wake up and tell myself today I'm going to eat right. Believe me I like donuts and chips like everybody else. My family and friends have given me a hard time over the years, making it seem as though it is very easy for me to stay thin. When strangers talk to me they say I must have good genes. I DON'T HAVE GOOD GENES! I have ok genes. I was one of five girls and you would think it would have been easy to eat right. But, my mother (whom is already deceased) was from Mexico and had a very traditional way of cooking, very rich high in calorie meals. Her and two of my four sisters are and were overweight my other two sisters are average. I am the only thin one. When I explain that I do have to work hard at staying slim they want to know how I do it. With that said I've become good at giving out advice on the subject I can only hope that it translates well into the written word. As a society we do a lot of over eating. It is hard to stay on track with all the eating out at restaurants, fast food, and family gatherings, not to mention all that processed food we eat and to top that off all the snacking we do to hold us over on busy days. THIS IS MY TAKE ON IT ALL!

In this short no nonsense easy to read and understand book I'll go over everything I do on a daily bases to stay healthy. Slim and trim is a bonus. I'll go over breakfast, lunch and dinner at home, juicing, eating out; fast food and restaurants, exercise, vitamins and last but not least snacking and desserts. That's where I'm going begin, with snacking and desserts. Sorry this is not a recipe book, but rather a book that will help you make your recipes a little healthier. You'll only find a few recipes in the book; some might seem like recipes but, they're more a how to on preparing some quick old faithful meals you make every day with a healthier twist on them.

The suggestions in this book are not intended to be a short term diet but as long term changes in the way you eat for the rest of your life. That is truly the only way it will work. You have to make smart choices on food and move a little.

DISCLAMER

If you or anyone in your family has allergies to any foods, milk, fruits, nuts or vitamins please continue to be careful with what you eat and anything you make like a juice. Labeling is a great way to indicate what is in a drink or pitcher. Please do not try anything your allergic to.

I would like to make it clear I am not endorsing any products or stores in this book. Simply letting you the readers know what I do and what I eat. I have taken pictures of products I buy to provide an example of the types of label you should be looking for and have posted them on social media, look for this book title. You may recognize some of these products. However it's to demonstrate what the fronts of these packages have on them such as calories, low fat or fat free. The name brand DOSE NOT MATTER.

If you are diabetic or are familiar with their diet it might seem at times like I eat like I'm diabetic. I do eat like I am, even thou I'm not, because it's smart to lower your sugar and carbohydrate intake. Many of the products sold nowadays that are sugar free taste good. This book is not intended for diabetics; if you are consult your doctor. Also keep in mind that too much salt isn't good for you and makes you retain fluids, there for a low salt diet is always a plus. As I said before I am not a dietitian, nutritionist or a doctor, just a house wife mother of four that has managed to keep off the pounds through the pregnancy's, the stress of life and the great high calorie food we're faced with every day.

SNACKING and DESSERST

I enjoy writing poetry so at the conclusion of this section I will leave you with a poem. I hope you enjoy it. It's about the world we live in now, a very fast pace, high stress world with so much to do and learn. Everyone is extremely busy these days and eating a snack because you're in a hurry is something we all get caught up in. Then there's also the snacking because the work day is dragging on, or the snack we get to enjoy a moment of eating something yummy we feel we deserve, that is everyone too, well at least everyone I know. Trying to staying away from chips and goodies is hard; I can't do it so I don't even try. I love chips with my sandwiches, just got to have something crunchy, and I love dessert. I do try hard not to let myself get too hungry so I don't over indulge in snacking. When I do need a snack I don't go buy a candy bar a bag of chips and a soda! Here's what I do.

Do for yourself what you do for your kids or what I hope you're doing for kids, pack a snack. Get the little snack size bags and fill them with heathy snacks and take them with you to work. On Saturday, buy some fruits and veggies like baby carrots, grapes and celery. Buy some dry items as well like nuts, pretzel, air pop popcorn and little boxes of raisins. For a woman, buy things you like that will travel well in your purse. For men things you could keep in your office or car. I hope you like raisins because they're really good for you and they'll cut the craving for sugar that we all get. Make sure you're not allergic to anything you buy like nuts. Fix them up on Saturday for the whole work week and leave them in the refrigerator ready to go, and leave the dry things on the counter easy to see and remember. I buy the big 32oz. bag of slivered almonds from the big national warehouse chain and cans of low salt mixed nuts and combine them. Other things you can buy for taking to work or to grab at home are the small containers of apple sauce, mandarin oranges, fat free gelatin or the fat free puddings. The puddings are my favorite. They're fat free and sugar free but, they do taste good.

When buying snacks or desserts for your home try the low calorie, fat free and sugar free products like ice cream and cookies. They're making them tastier these days. You may have to try different brands of cookies some taste better than others. Even the not so great ones will taste good with a cup of coffee. If its cake time at a party or at home take off most the frosting and get a small slice. Enjoy all other desserts like donuts or a slice of pie, one or the other, every few days not every day. Never deprive yourself. We Americans need to take a page from the French, eating your dessert moderately and slowly, take the time to enjoy the taste of what we're eating. If you diet, by passing up desserts, snacks and eating small meals you'll run out of energy. This can lower your immune system making it easier to catch a cold and the flu among other things. Not really a healthy thing to do. The following is a quick health dessert:

Strawberry Chill

1 box vanilla wafers about 40 cookies

3 cups flavored yogurt

3 cups of strawberries frozen (thawed) or fresh

4 teaspoons sweetener (sucralose, stevia, or sugar)

1 can light whip topping (optional)

Line a casserole dish with wafers. It will take about 20. Then smooth 1 ½ cup yogurt over the cookies. You can add a little sweetener to the yogurt, like 1 to2 teaspoons sucralose, stevia or sugar. In a separate bowl mix strawberries with 1 tablespoon sugar. Take ½ of the strawberries and spread over yogurt. Repeat with a second layer then cover with plastic or foil and refrigerate overnight. Top individual servings with whip cream and enjoy. I like to buy the light yogurts with only 100 calories with the fruit on the bottom, you can also buy reduce fat vanilla wafers. If you do, each 2 inch by 2 inch square of dessert is about 100 calories.

Destine

This planet so big and vast

Our lives and times are moving fast

So much to learn

And I do yearn

To know what makes it

And what shapes it

As I look around

And hear the sounds

Of all the things that move me

From the trees to the seas

Suddenly

I know its ok

I know it in my heart

I'm bound to be a part

By Magalene Y. Noble

BREAKFAST

Many people like to skip breakfast, if at all possible don't do that. It is said that it's the most important meal of the day. I'm not sure about that but, I do know eating several small meals throughout the day is better for you than eating one or two large meals. The smaller meals can digest easier and will keep your stomach from becoming too larger. If your stomach gets too large it will take more food to fill it and as soon as you cut back or change how you eat you'll feel hungry.

Breakfast can be tricky, I do eat eggs but I don't eat the yoke. I make the eggs over medium and eat around the yoke trying not to break it. It might seem silly but you have to keep in mind it is all the little things that you do that add up to big results. The yoke is the fatty part of the egg and the white part is the protein. I don't eat pork for the most part no bacon no sausage. I know, boo. You can try the turkey bacon. An egg meal for me would consist of two eggs over medium, two table spoons fat free cottage cheese or refried beans and a slice of toast. If you really like the yoke or don't think you'll get full off two eggs without the yoke make yourself three eggs but only eat one of the yoke.

I do eat cold and hot cereal. When buying cold cereal choose one that is multigrain low sugar one of my favorite is bran flakes with raisins and I use fat free or skim milk. If you don't drink that kind of milk already it will take a little getting accustom to, start with 2% then switch to 1% after a few months then to fat free after a year. If you just can't do it at least you're drinking 1% and that's not bad. I really like oatmeal and it does give you that good full feeling. Get the quick oats you have to cook on the stove it just taste better than instant, and don't buy the flavored kind it has a lot of sugar and calories. When cooking your oatmeal use less of the oats then it calls for then add a little milk so that it's not too thick, sweeten with your choice of sweeteners, I use stevia. When done add one table spoon slivered almonds and one table spoon cranberries (craisins) or raisins. (If you're not allergic to nuts, cranberries or raisins) Don't have toast bread, if you do, eat less of the oatmeal.

Pancakes, waffles and French toast are breakfast items that don't seem there's any way for them to be healthy but where there's a will there's a way. Let's talk pancakes, make your batter any brand add two cups of fruit for every four servings you mix up. Don't be afraid it will cook up just fine. When I add bananas I smash one really well and anther I leave chunky add both to the batter. Smash another to add to the top after they're cooked. Use very little light syrup, and no butter. Waffles, simple I buy the multi grain low fat ones they taste great and you can't tell the difference, again add fruit to top or just have fruit on the side. French toast is my favorite and the easiest to make healthy. For a serving of three or four, crack three eggs into a bowl adding only the egg whites and one whole egg. Then 2 ½ cups of 1% or fat free milk, three tea spoons sweetener of choice and cinnamon. Use whole wheat bread if you can eat wheat. Cook on a griddle using a canola spray, should yield about 8 pieces. Top with a little light syrup.

Before I end breakfast let me just say I add slivered almonds to everything I eat for breakfast. I add one tablespoon to my cereal hot and cold I put one tablespoon on the top of my pancakes, waffles and French toast. As you know these breakfast items don't have much too any protein. This adds a little much needed protein. When I'm in a hurry I get a slice of bread and put one teaspoon peanut butter two teaspoons cocoa hazelnut spread on it and sprinkle one tablespoon slivered almonds in the middle. I do have a yogurt and a slice of toast for breakfast sometimes; I get the light 100 calorie or less Greek yogurts with fruit on the bottom. Let's not forget your morning cup of coffee; this is where you can really feel that you started the day out right. Use a little bit of milk and a little bit of fat free creamer or a fat free and sugar free creamer then a little bit of a sugar substitute.

LUNCH

When preparing lunch for yourself to eat at home or to take on the go the only thing you need to take in consideration is time. Do you have time to cook some thing or are you just making a sandwich or a burrito. If you don't have time or just don't want to spend too much time preparing lunch you need to have items there in place to keep it low calorie and healthy.

The items I keep on hand are; 97% fat free ham, tuna, cans of ranch beans, tomato, avocado, romaine lettuce, frozen peas, fat free cottage cheese, and light salad dressing spread. Other items you will need bread or flour tortillas, hot sauce and salsa.

Here's how you bring all these items together in different meals. A tuna sandwich; mix one can of tuna with 2 teaspoons light salad dressing spread and 1 cup cooked frozen peas a little salt and pepper spread on bread, top with another. (If you don't usually use light salad dressing spread, give it a try it has more flavor than mayonnaise and you will have to use less of it, I do get the name brand of that product.) Let's make a low calorie burrito or lettuce wrap. Heat up a flour tortilla (A small 8" round) or a wedge of romaine lettuce put one slice of lean sandwich ham, ¼ avocado, 3 teaspoons ranch beans (heated and smashed, don't refried them), 3 teaspoons fat free cottage cheese, a little hot sauce or salsa (salsa can be a life saver it makes most everything taste great, and is good for you too, give it a try.) I have included a recipe for my salsa in the recipe section.

DINNER

Let me start with a salad, it's my favorite meal. The amount you use of each item would be based on how many people are going to eat and what you like. Wash some lettuce, spinach, tomatoes, shredded carrots and toss in a large bowl. Sprinkle top with craisins, slivered almonds, and sliced strawberries. Use your favorite dressing to finish it off. I like to use raspberry balsamic vinaigrette. You can add some grilled chicken or some roasted chicken you bought already cooked from your big national warehouse chain store to make it a complete dinner.

Did I say chicken, how many different ways can we make chicken? My answer let me count the ways.

1. Chicken Cacciatore

2. Chicken Tostadas

3. Chicken Enchiladas

4. Chicken stir fry Lettuce wrap

5. Grilled Chicken and Mashed potatoes

6. Barb B Q Chicken

7. Baked Chicken and Mushrooms

8. Green Chile Chicken Casserole

9. Chicken Salad

10. Chicken and Rice soup

Do you have more? If you do that's great. I don't get tiered of chicken but you have to change up the meals you make out of it. Here are the things you need to know to make all your recipes a little healthier. When cooking your meals if you're going to use oil use a blend of light olive oil and canola. The olive oil has just as many calories as the canola but it is better for you and doesn't turn into stored fat as easy. I do recommend the light olive oil it doesn't have as rich of a flavor as the extra virgin olive oil. Don't use too much cheese in your recipes. Cheese is a dairy product but is high in fat. Try reduced fat cheese products they do work the same in your dishes and taste good. I do like to eat a lot of other meals as well like fish, spaghetti, lasagna, Swiss steak, e.c.t. But I make a salad or server myself fat free cottage cheese along with plenty of vegetables that were made with the meal. Always make vegetables with your meals. On taco night or with a Mexican meal slice tomatoes and put a little olive oil, lemon, pepper and salt, lay the tomatoes over chopped lettuce. With your Italian foods pizza, lasagna and spaghetti make a salad and some baby carrots or broccoli. Teaching your children to eat and like there vegetables is the best thing you can do for their health. If there is something they don't like, broccoli for instance, try putting cheese on it better a little cheese then no vegies. If they don't like carrots add a little sweetener. A Swiss steak (Swiss steak is cubed thin steak cooked with tomatoes, onion and bell pepper) dinner plate would be 2 tablespoons of Swiss steak over 3 tablespoons rice 3 tablespoons of frozen peas cooked or steamed and 1 tablespoon fat free cottage cheese.

RECIPES

Here are a few recipes from the list of chicken dinners.

Chicken Tostadas

3 pieces chicken breast

10 corn tortillas

¼ cup light olive oil, combined with ¼ cup canola oil

3 tomatoes

1 small yellow onion

1 teaspoon salt

1 teaspoon pepper

2 cups shredded lettuce

1 cup reduced fat shredded cheddar cheese

1 can ranch style beans (smashed) or 1 can pinto beans (smashed)

Boil chicken with ½ teaspoon salt and ½ teaspoon pepper; once fully cooked allow the chicken to cool, then shred. Dice two tomatoes and the onion and cook in a large skillet for about five minutes. Add the shredded chicken to the tomatoes and onions. Mix well and add more salt and pepper if needed. Continue to cook for five minutes and remove from heat and set aside. Now were ready to make the fried corn tortillas. Make sure you have tongs as you will have to flip the tortillas as they cook. In a small skillet heat oil blend on medium heat, once hot, fry the corn tortillas until golden brown and crisp. Be careful with the hot oil it tends to splash when hot and could cause a fire if it falls on stove and comes in contact with fire. Make sure the oil level does not exceed half –way up the skillet so it does not spill when putting the tortilla in the oil. If the oil gets low you can add a little more. Cook all ten one at a time taking very good care not to burn them. They do cook fast and may bubble up. Remove the bubbles by press out with fork. You can buy them in the grocery store already made but, they don't taste as good as the ones you make at home. In another small skillet heat up beans, until hot and mash them up. Slice or dice up the remaining tomato and put in small bowl and set aside. On the fried corn tortilla spread 1 tablespoon of beans, then spread 1 tablespoon chicken on top of beans. Top with shredded lettuce cheese and a few slices of tomato. If you like hot sauce or salsa it will taste great on the tostadas. That's a real touch of Mexico! Hope you enjoy. Serves about four to five

Chicken and Rice Soup

3 pieces chicken breast

½ teaspoon salt

½ teaspoon pepper

½ pound bag baby carrots

½ cup rice

¾ cup frozen peas

½ jalapeño deseeded (optional)

1 tablespoon cilantro (optional)

1 lime (optional)

Cube the chicken and boil with salt and pepper in five quart pot or bigger, cook for thirty minutes. Then half the carrots and add to the pot, cooking an additional thirty minutes. Add peas to the pot, (frozen is fine) cooking ten more minutes. Then add the uncooked rice, cooking until rice is tender. It should take about fifteen, twenty minutes for rice to be done. You can easily give this soup a Mexican flare by adding half a deseeded jalapeño to the soup when you put it to boil. Then add 1 table spoon of cilantro to the soup when you add the carrots. Finish with adding a twist of lime to your bowl. Try it both ways. Either way I'm sure you will enjoy this quick, easy- to- make soup. Serves about four to five

Salsa

3 tomatoes

1 small onion or ½ a large one

3 tablespoons cilantro

2 cloves of garlic

1 or 2 jalapeños (depending on how spicy you want it)

1 to 2 cups of water

1 teaspoon chicken bouillon

1 teaspoon salt

2 tablespoons light olive oil

Dice tomatoes, onion, cilantro, jalapeño and garlic. Blend everything together with 1 cup of water for thirty seconds. Add the chicken bouillon, blend until everything is well blended, taste for salt and add water, add as needed, shouldn't be too thick. In medium size skillet heat oil until hot. Pour mixture into pan, be careful oil will splash; fry until tomatoes turn a darker red this should take about ten minutes to be done.

Chicken Salad

3 pieces chicken breast

½ cup frozen peas

1 cup shredded carrots

1 cup lettuce

2 tablespoons light salad dressing spread

½ teaspoon salt

½ teaspoon pepper

Boil chicken with salt and pepper, cool and shred. Once cooled add peas, carrots and lettuce. Then add the salad dressing spread and stir. Serves about four to five

FAST FOOD and RESTAURANTS

Fast food, we all have to do it from time to time some more than others. If you're a busy family you're probably doing it often. I know making the right choices are hard and it gets boring but that really is the only way to keep the pounds off. Yes, I'm going to say it order grilled chicken on wheat if possible hold the mayo or ask for very little mayo sometimes they put too much, better to little than too much. Have them add tomato and lettuce if it doesn't come with it. Don't get the French fries. Don't drink soda. None sweeten tea (use stevia or sucralose to sweeten or ask for the little packets of sugar for your drink the sweetened tea has a lot of sugar far more than the 3 packets you might add for a large tea) or best of all get water. Some fast food places will let you replace the fries with other healthier items, it doesn't hurt to ask. You're going to order the hamburger; I know chicken gets old, get the small one and have them add lettuce, tomato and onions if it doesn't come with it. Order the side salad with low fat, reduced fat, or fat free dressing. If it doesn't taste good to you add pepper and a little salt or go with regular balsamic vinaigrette. All the little things you do throughout the day add up and it will add up to a smaller waist if you stick to it.

Off to the restaurant on a dinner date or just a business lunch. No matter which, here's how to handle it. Order meals that are cooked with plenty of vegetables, if that is not an option, and then order a bowl of broccoli, stemmed carrots on the side or a side salad, and eat at all your vegies. Ask for all sauces and dressing on the side, and use them moderately. My self personally I don't eat much red meat I eat fish and chicken, If you are going to order steak, whether a male or female, get a small one 6 oz. Brisket and steak are harder for your stomach to digest. At the same time you place the order ask for a too go box. When your plate comes, before you start to eat, put ½ to ¼ of your plate into the box use your own judgment. But I can guaranty its more food than you need or even want. If you're going back to work and don't have any were to store it give it to a co-worker I'm sure there's always someone that had to work thru lunch just let them know you put it in the box before you ate any of it. Do that a few times and they'll take you out to lunch unless, you're the boss. When I'm out with family or a good friend I order my own side salad or cup of soup, yes cup not a bowl, then we share the entrée. Some restaurants charge for the extra plate, look for the ones that don't, some will gladly split it up for you in the kitchen at no charge. If you find yourself at the all you can eat buffet start with a salad. When I make my salad I like to get the darker greens and some sunflower seeds I never put cheese, bacon bits or croutons on my salad. Serve yourself plenty of vegetables and stay moderate on the meat and dessert. Keep in mind that if you over eat too often it will continue take more food to feel full. Enjoy!

JUICING

Juicing is the best way to a get power dose of fiber and natural vitamins and yes I do it. Here are the hints you need to do it the smart way, you'll find it very easy and economical. Don't go out and buy an expensive juicing machine, I tried it. Yes there easy to use, but not so easy to clean and you really do throw away a lot of good healthy fiber. At the end of the day you will get tiered of buying pounds of vegetables for the tiny amount of juice you get. There are also high powered blenders you can buy that are great for juicing the whole vegetable, but you don't need one of those either your regular blender is all you need.

There are different kinds of drinks I make all of them contain spinach. The good thing about spinach is that when you blend it with other foods like bananas it has very little to no taste. I really didn't know this but a good friend of mine told me to try it. Not a problem for me I really love spinach and eat it often, but the traditional way blanched with a little vinegar, yummy. So this was a great way to add more fruits and vegetables to my diet. I try to drink a glass a day every day but if I can't I do Monday thru Friday and if I miss a day or two during the week I will make that effort to drink one on the week end. Don't be afraid to go green!

I buy the large 16 oz. container of organic baby spinach and the large 52 oz. bottle of organic carrot juice from a large national warehouse chain. The only bad thing about spinach is that it doesn't have a long shelve life. You will have to use the container within five days or so. Play around with different variations. You can always substitute the apple juice for carrot juice or the carrot juice for orange juice and so forth. Try making your own passion fruit juice. You will have to peel, cut and wash all the fruit. So with that said, don't do it too often or you will want to quit. We live in a fast pace busy world so keeping it simple is key to continued success. If you or any one in your house hold has allergies to any fruits or vegetables please make sure you are careful. You might want to label the cups or containers. Another thing you have to do to keep it simple is wash the blender immediately after use .If the spinach dries it's like concrete. If you don't have time to wash the blender, rinse it out well. If this is something you don't think you would like to do don't stress over it. I am fifty two years old and have only been doing this for one year; there are plenty of things in the book that are very helpful and are the things I have done most my life.

Here are some combinations you need to try;

4 oz. of apple juice

1 banana- broken into four pieces

2 to 4 oz. water

2 cups loosely packed spinach (all combinations will contain 1 or 2 cups of spinach. Make sure you wash the spinach thoroughly.

Put the banana into the blender first, add the apple juice, then add the water and loosely packed spinach to the blender slowly. Blend on pulse or chop for the first few seconds then liquefy until spinach is well blended. Pure over ice, you can add the ice to blender but I don't recommend this, it will dull the blade.

4 oz. of carrot juice

1 small tomato

1 apple peeled, cored and cut into 6 pieces

1 cup loosely packed spinach

2 to 4 oz. water

Put the tomato and apples in the blender first add the carrot juice and spinach same as before, pulse then liquefy add water as needed to blend.

Treat yourself to a sweet healthy dessert

½ cup strawberries frozen or fresh

½ cup blueberries frozen or fresh

1 teaspoon sweetener, sugar, sucralose or stevia

4 oz. apple juice

2 to 4 oz. of water

1 cups, loosely packed spinach

1 cup crush ice

1 -5oz, container of Greek yogurt with fruit (If you can't eat dairy substitute with what you can drink; like silk milk, almond milk or lactose free milk)

Blend fruit and spinach first with apple juice, sweetener and water then the add yogurt and ice. Add sweetener to taste.

VITAMINS

Where do I stand on the vitamin issue? I take them, I can only speak for myself but I did feel a difference when I started taking a multivitamin regularly, the key word here is regularly. I have been taking vitamins off and on for most my life but, there were times I didn't take any vitamins for years. In 1998 I was in a car accident and I had an x- ray of my spine. I was fine from the accident but the doctor said I should start taking calcium because he could see some deterioration of the bone in my spinal Colom, most likely from carrying my children. I was about 36 years old at that time. I have been taking calcium ever since, but I won't lie it took me years to get in the habit of taking a pill every day and even now I forget sometimes that I should take it twice a day. The good thing is I make sure the multivitamin I take has calcium as well. Please consult your doctor before starting any vitamin regimen, especially if you are taking any medications even vitamins and herbs can have adverse reactions with some medications.

I do buy a good multivitamin now from a well-known vitamin store, Yes, a little pricy. I get the ones that are especially made for senior women and are time release. I did work up to taking those; I started with taking a regular generic multivitamin about 13, 14 years ago when I was 38, 39, then a generic multivitamin for seniors, 5 years later when I was 45. At 50 I started taking the time release vitamin.

The complete vitamin regimen I'm on is as follows;(don't get scared, it sounds like a lot more than it is) Calcium -twice a day, multivitamin- once a day, omga-3 fish oil- twice a day, flaxseed oil -twice a day. Read the dosing instructions and take them as directed. I keep it all organized in the medication containers that are for a week, I have one for the morning and one for the afternoon.

EXERCISE

I know, it's not bad enough we have to eat right we have to exercise also. The good news is if you eat right you don't have to kill yourself exercising. I have been thin most of my life with the exception of coarse throughout my pregnancies. When I was young I did like to run and bike ride, something I kept up through high school. Eating right was also something I always attempted off and on through the years as with everything sometimes it was harder than others. It still is now, but over the years I have looked for ways to make both eating right and exercising a little easier.

Before I start talking about my exercise routines let me just say I do the little things that add up when it comes to exercise as well. I take the stairs instead of the elevator. If I'm not in a hurry I park at the back of the parking lot. Try not to pass up opportunities where you can get a little extra exercise in, Make sure that you have the ok to exercise from your doctor.

It is hard to exercise! It's hard to find the time and energy, especially at the same time. For that reason I try to it keep quick and simple. I change up what I do; no, not the routine at the gym, the routine I do from one day to another. I try not to let myself get bored. One day I'll go for a long walk and work out a little at home. The next day I'll just work out at home. The following day I'll go for a short brisk walk and a short work out at home. Yes, I do go to the gym intermittently. I do have to admit it I find it hard to get there sometimes even if I have the time. However, I do enjoy the workout I get there so I do try to go. On a busy day If I find the day light getting away from me and there's no time for a walk or a good work out at home I do a quick work out on my trouble spots, waist, stomach and inner thighs.

Workouts I do at home are not too long or complicated. I started with side stretches. I do about fifty to one hundred depending on if the plan is a long or short work out. Leg lifts to the side in the standing position, two reps of twenty. I do twenty pushups on the wall or holding the counter top. Move your hips in circular motion with your hands on them to the count of fifty. I do have an ab scissor I use I do 3 reps of twenty. Most of the exercise I do I started at ten or twenty first. If you don't have anything to work your abs out with do sit ups on your bed. Start with 3 reps of 5. You can do leg lifts on your bed as well laying on your side 3 reps of 5 on both sides. The leg lifts will work out your sides too. Don't overdo it start at a low number and work up increasing by five or ten. When doing reps do only three reps of ten and start to increase. The same applies for the gym. Start with low weight and do three reps of five or ten slowly start to increase the weight and continue to do three reps but increase the number. For example if you were doing three reps of five do three reps of ten. Don't rush to increase weights or the number in the reps. Increase weights after a week or two. If you feel more comfortable after a month that is fine, the best way to do it is slow. If you end up to sore the chances are higher you'll stop going. Or stop working out even if at home.

CONCULSION

When I said short I meant it! I would like to apologize for the length. I felt it was important to be short and to the point and leave out the fluff, also for any poor grammar you might have had to endure. I just have a few more things I would like to add. I don't talk about calorie counting, but that was intentional losing weight is a numbers game calories in, calories out but if you make some good choices throughout the day there's no need to get bogged down with that. There's one important thing you want to look at carefully when looking at the nutrition label on the side of packages and that's how many servings it's for. Often when you buy small drinks or bags of chips that look like single servings it might be two or three servings so you have to double or triple the calories. If you are someone that could benefit from my advice but feel these small changes won't help .Don't sell yourself short, give it a try. I know some of you probably think it would take forever to lose the weight making these changes, but always keep in mind it took time to put on the weight and if you take your time losing it, you will keep the weight off. I would also like to remind you that the advice I give in this book is not intended for the short term but as a lifelong change.

Change is hard but the changes you make when it comes to food will change everything. You will be healthier, you will think clearer, you will have more energy, and you'll live longer. If you have to start in phases do that, but do it. I would like to thank you for the opportunity to come into your life for a brief moment and share what I do with you. I sincerely hope it works for you.